A SUPER Home
Exercise Book
For Seniors

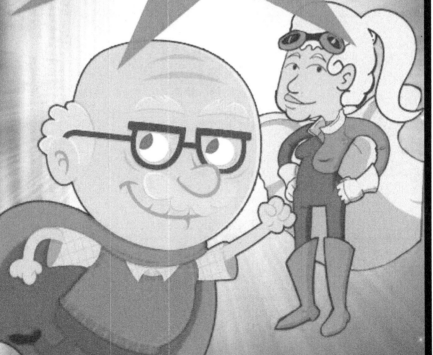

Kevin Saint Clair

Best Sellers in Exercise & Fitness For the Aging

1. LOOK INSIDE!

Core Strength for 50+: A
Customized P...
by Karl Knopf
☆☆☆☆☆ ☑ (15)
Paperback
$12.58
30 used & new from $9.31

2. LOOK INSIDE!

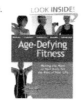

Age Defying Fitness: Making
the Most...
by Marilyn Moffat
☆☆☆☆☆ ☑ (36)
Paperback
$16.25
51 used & new from $10.00

3. LOOK INSIDE!

Somatics: Reawakening
The Mind's Cont...
by Thomas Hanna
☆☆☆☆☆ ☑ (80)
Paperback
$14.82
86 used & new from $10.23

4. LOOK INSIDE!

Cycling Past 50 (Ageless
Athlete)
by Joe Friel

5. LOOK INSIDE!

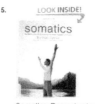

Somatics: Reawakening
The Mind's Cont...
by Thomas Hanna

6. LOOK INSIDE!

A SUPER Home Exercise
Book for Senior...
by Kevin Saint Clair - Home

"Thank you to everyone around the world who made this book an international best seller on Amazon.

This book is my FREE GIFT TO YOU this holiday season, to help you increase your strength while at home, or wherever you may be, in hopes that it makes your 2016...SUPER!

Never give up. ☺"

- Kevin Saint Clair
The Frisco Consulting Group

Special Note: Please consult your physician before you begin this or any other exercise program. If at any point, you feel pain or shortness of breath, stop immediately and consult your physician.

Enjoy!

Table of Contents

DEDICATION

This book is dedicated to my late Uncle,

Stanley Hodkinson, a.k.a. "Uncle Stan."

Uncle Stan had a tremendous amount of positive energy and a passion for living. He did his best to pass that on to "us kids" many years ago. Uncle Stan was successful in his mission. I want to thank Uncle Stan for the love, joy and determination that he left as a legacy.

Chapter 1

Why This Routine Is SUPER Effective

Your muscles are directly connected to the Central Nervous System of the body. Among other duties, your Central Nervous System controls how your body is designed to adapt from external stimuli.

The process of getting stronger is simply cause & effect.

What makes the routine in this book more effective, in terms of gaining strength, than the methods espoused by most conventional magazines is this:

In order to send the safest, most efficient signal to your body and tell it to become stronger, you must not only avoid the weak (and most dangerous) range of motion (which every exercise possesses) but also push the targeted muscle, safely, in it's strongest range of motion and do so in a manner that is required, to send a specific signal to your central nervous system which causes this "trigger" to take place. This is a simple, yet specialized process.

Most exercise routines will have you doing repetitions of 10, or 15, or some arbitrary number and suggest that you stop at the certain number.

After studying this science for almost 25 years, I can tell you that these numbers are of "stone age" mentality and there is a much faster and safer way for you to manipulate this aspect of your central nervous system.

The routine in this book is a very good starting point for anyone, but I chose this routine and it's introductory level of exercises to benefit Seniors FIRST.

On occasion and with certain clients, I get a little more in-depth, with more progressive, scientific explanations, beyond what I explain here. However, this routine is a great starting point to anyone with any number of "loss-of-strength" conditions.

This initial routine is much more efficient and effective in helping a senior regain their strength, than many other routines, which provide extremely outdated exercise advice and often leaves readers doing endless routines, consisting of sub-par exercises. And grasping at straws to feel results.

Start with the routine in this book. Start today!

It's as simple as getting a tan.

For example, when you spend time out in the sun, your central nervous system releases a chemical called melanin. Melanin travels to the skin and begins the process of causing the skin to become darker.

The longer or more intense the sun's exposure, the more chemicals are released into the blood stream and the darker (or redder) the skin becomes.

People who lay on beaches with the desire to develop a tan are simply **manipulating this process of self-preservation.**
It is very simple. The process of getting in shape is much simpler than most magazines would have you believe.

Bright Lights!

Another example of this wonderful adaptation process we all possess is when the pupils of the eye are subjected to a bright light, they constrict or shrink in order to protect sensitive nerves from incurring any damage from the applied "stress" (bright light).

These only are two examples of the amazing self-preservation system that our bodies are equipped with, since the days of the cavemen (and camerawomen) to handle many of the stressors of the outside world. The muscles of the body respond in exactly the same manner, if given the proper signals to do so.

Does the information start to make sense now?

The process of how a callous is formed on the hands is the EXACT same process, but I think you get the idea.

In a nutshell, these features of our Central Nervous System work sort of like this…

First, an outside stress is applied and then our bodies are forced to adapt. Depending on the severity or simplicity of the stress, this adaptation could occur immediately (pupils) or, in the case of a burn, it could take days (or even weeks in severe cases). There are many different processes occurring during the healing and adapting phases, inside the body, but for the sake of this book and to stick to the point, it works like this…

STRESS…
ADAPT…
STRESS…
ADAPT.

· The exercises contained in this book and the manner in which I have you perform them are only the triggers which cause the stress.

The next 24-48 hours will allow for the adaptation process to take place.

I hope you understand how simple this process is. There will NOT be a quiz at the end of the book.

Who likes quizzes?

Not me!

Our Bodies are in a Natural State of Decline

Research has shown that in the fourth decade of life, the muscle mass of the human body starts to decrease annually by three to five percent.

This means most men and women begin to see a decline in muscle strength and muscle mass beginning in our 40s, although lack of exercise, poor diet, injuries or just sitting around can also cause you to lose valuable muscle.
Your body needs this muscle. Your skeleton is supported by muscle. Without strong muscle tissue throughout your body, you literally begin to slowly wither away. There have been many studies showing the effects in-action has on muscle tissue.

Suffice to say that **doing nothing is in fact doing something**. Doing nothing allows your body to deteriorate.

This physical decline of our bodies continues throughout the remainder of our lives and is directly responsible for a loss of agility, strength, flexibility and mobility which can get worse and worse as time goes on.

Losing these important aspects of physical health, has often been related to depression, loneliness and feeling withdrawn. You or someone you love may be affected by these negative conditions right now.

Our Pain

Millions of Americans suffer from back and joint pain every day — much of this pain is CAUSED by weak-supporting muscles. As a result, millions of Americans are prescribed and take billions of pills each day to "mask" the pain.

The truth is, taking medications for pain does nothing to address the problem and in fact can cause a host of other problems in the body such as dependency, liver & kidney failure and even overdose and death. The deaths caused by accidental prescription pill overdose in America are shocking.

According to the Center for Disease Control, overdoses involving prescription painkillers are at epidemic levels and now kill more Americans than heroin and cocaine combined.

We are an over-indulgent society and our relatively new consumption of massive amounts of pain pills is no exception.

There are many people who have sustained injuries, and medications for the pain are necessary.

However, I feel most people also would like to address the root of the problem (when it is caused by weak muscles) so they may only have to take these medications on an as-needed basis.

It is my hope that if we can help each other with knowledge, which helps loved ones develop a happier, healthier body. It is important that we are proud of the body we "own."

As concerned citizens, we should be able to share this type of information with people who need it the most. The goal is together, we may be able to assist MANY people affected with negative, hopeless thoughts and replace them with laughter, zest and a **greater sense of LIFE!**

Why I Wrote This Book

I wrote this book in hopes of equipping you, the senior, with some tools you can use, at home, in order to help improve your strength, mobility and perhaps ease some of your physical pain.

Your quality of life gradually becomes acted-upon by the aging process. We all have been known to get comfortable at some point in our lives with our diet and physical activity. However, we all know full well that time stops for no man (or woman) and each day that passes without taking action, to re-gain our strength and mobility is one more day we simply cannot get back.

Time is one of our most precious commodities in life. Everyone should cherish time. One should use time as motivation to fuel your fire each day. This book is designed to be a tool in your fight against the aging process. I am a firm believer that if a person has the sheer will and desire to change their lifestyle and habits, anything is possible.

This book, though primarily a "Beginner's Guide" to regaining or maintaining your strength, is only a small portion of exercise methods I use to assist people to help them regain and increase their strength. There are more advanced exercises (some requiring basic equipment) to help develop the strength in every muscle of the body. I wanted to first provide you with some basic but highly effective movements you can do in the privacy of your own home.

Hopefully, this routine helps to improve your quality of life.

Foreword

The group of exercises listed in this book will be enough to get you started on the road to being a stronger "you." It will also hopefully help reduce or eliminate some back, shoulder or other joint pain, which is suffered by millions of people every day.

Please feel free to pass this link on to a friend, family member or neighbor.

Together, we truly can make a difference!

Uncle Stan

One of my inspirations as a kid (and for wanting to help others) was my Uncle Stan. Uncle Stan lived in Cumberland, Rhode Island. Growing up in Virginia, we used to travel up to Rhode Island and visit our extended family.

Uncle Stan was a "man's man." He was the guy in our family who used to say to us kids "Go ahead, punch me in the stomach." Uncle Stan was in his 60s and spent each morning in his basement exercising with free weights and his punching bag.

He also had a speed bag set up and was eager to show us how to us one properly (think Rocky Balboa). Uncle Stan had a heart of gold and was as tough as they come. — at least to us kids. He always was smiling, full of energy and used to run around with us kids, in the backyard, when we would go up north to visit.

Uncle Stan made a very positive impact on me as a child. He stressed the importance of keeping ourselves in shape. He enjoyed different types of food, desserts and snacks in moderation. Uncle Stan knew how important it was to keep his physical self healthy & strong.

He always said "I'm not gonna grow old gracefully…I'm gonna go down fighting!" The guy had class. It was a joy and pleasure to be able to learn from him.

While you certainly do not have to use a punching bag every day, doing some type of exercise daily translates into having better, USEABLE strength and has also be proven to:

Increase self-esteem

Fight depression

Increase metabolism

Increase lean muscle tissue

DECREASE body fat

Reduce or eliminate chronic pain

Reduce your dependence on certain types of drugs

Improve your quality of life and...

Allow you to play with your grandchildren more!

The benefits of getting (and keeping) your body in better shape, goes on and on!

The SUPER Convenience of This Routine

One of the great aspects of this workout is that you can literally begin doing it RIGHT NOW.

You do not have to get dressed and go to a health club. It does not matter what you are wearing. There are no fashion police to worry about!

Another great time to begin this routine is the moment you wake up in the morning.

The time you begin this routine is up to you, so long as you START DOING IT. Remember that doing nothing is in fact doing something to your body. We get weaker and weaker each day we decide to NOT take action. We can tell our bodies to get stronger and better.

Do not let another day go by and allow nature to keep "having her way with you."

Get excited about making this positive change in your life.

Make up your mind to take control of your body, your strength and your happiness and do it today!

Chapter 2

Getting Started

This book will teach you some of the basic methods I have used to assist people in regaining their strength and mobility.

Ultimately, making the decision to fight the aging process and attempt to develop a better quality of life for yourself will have to be your decision.

You will have to be the one to look at your current level of mobility, fitness, obesity, health and mindset and say to yourself...

"I want to move better, feel better and LIVE BETTER!"

The human body is an amazingly resilient creation. If it is given the correct signals to grow stronger and get better, it is miraculous what it is able to overcome.

Believe me when I tell you the results are worth it.

Use It or Lose It

Our muscles fall into the "use it or lose it" category. The good news is that much of what you have lost, YOU CAN GET BACK.

What you may not know, however, is that it's is simple for you to regain the strength, agility and mobility you possessed many years ago. Some people I assisted over the years and after months of personal one-on-one sessions with me, seniors have been able to discontinue the use of certain types of medication for pain, high cholesterol and others.

I want to stress that I am NOT a physician. I simply am someone who has a passion for learning a few things about the functions of the human body, and also someone who has spent the past couple of decades researching and applying much of what I have learned.

I have a tremendous amount of respect for the great people who dedicate their lives providing medical care to all of us for each of our conditions.

You will be doing some of the most effective exercises possible to begin to strengthen some of the major muscles of the body.

You will be able to do these in the comfort of your own home.

The Big 3

In the interest of keeping this book fun and informative without diving into every single muscle group in your body, I am going to mention a very important group of muscles.

I like to call this group "**The Big 3**."

The Lower Back

The muscles of the lower back known as the spinal erector (or erector spinae) muscles are responsible for controlling the movement around the base of your spine. As the name implies, they erect your spine from a lying or seated position.

They consist of two muscles that run up and down either side of your spine. These muscles are certainly one of the most important muscle groups in your body.

Therefore, they need to be strengthened and KEPT STRONG at all times in order for you to be able to function to the best of your ability. Without these muscles acting in their strong "supporting" role (for which they are designed), the rest of the muscles of your upper torso and lower body become increasingly difficult to control. Simply put, you can possess strong shoulders, arms, legs, or all of the above, but if your lower back muscles are weak, you are at prime risk of (or perhaps have already had) a painful injury of the lower back.

Remember the Straw Man in The Wizard of OZ?

He was always falling to one side and then to the other. They had to keep propping him up!

Granted, he did not even have a spine, but I think you get the idea.

My point is to stress how important it is to maintain the strength in the muscles of the lower back — though he did possess some rather interesting dance moves!

The Upper Back

The upper back muscles allow us to sit up, stand up and roll over. (dogs have great upper back muscles). However, one thing we can do, which dogs cannot (sorry Fido) is pick things up.

Without strong upper back muscles, we must rely on others to lift and carry things for us. Let's be honest…that is just not fun. As inevitable as it may be for all of us to rely on others for certain things, we speed up the process. If we want to regain and maintain our strength, (and certain aspects of our independence) **we must strengthen the muscles of the upper back.**

The Muscles Of The "rear end."

Your gluteus maximus or "glutes" are the largest muscle group on the body.

They are one of the muscles that are responsible for allowing you to get out of bed each day (and out of your chair.)

A comparison I like to draw in order to convey the importance of this muscle group is simply taking a look at the ostrich…

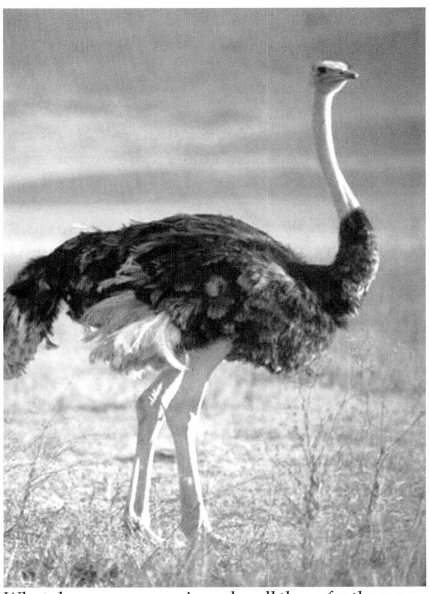

What do you suppose is under all those feathers on the ostrich's rear end?

What do you think he's hiding under there?

I'll tell you…it's **MUSCLE!**

Now, do not be afraid of looking like an ostrich as you begin to strengthen your "rear end" (you also won't become one of the fastest creatures on earth) but to an ostrich, the "glutes" are as important as survival itself.

Without those strong glutes to move around…the poor ostrich would not be able to run after or AWAY from anything.

(Now some of you can tell your friends that you learned something from an ostrich today.)
☺

Chapter 4

This exercise routine should be performed once per day for three days a week for four weeks.

Due to the nature of how your central nervous system functions, it is recommended that your first routine be performed on a Monday-Wednesday-Friday schedule. This is my recommendation for the routine in this book. An alternative schedule would be a Saturday-Monday-Wednesday schedule.

The main point is that you do your first routine on Day 1, and then you allow your body a rest day to recover and become stronger from the previous routine.

One should perform the routine on the following day, rest the next day and then the third and final workout of the week should be performed on the following day thereafter.

After three consecutive workouts, you should then give your body two days of rest (walking) and begin the routine again in the same manner the following week.

Your new Home 30 day exercise routine should look like this...

Monday - Exercise
Tuesday - Walk
Wednesday - Exercise
Thursday - Walk
Friday - Exercise
Saturday - Walk
Sunday – Rest

Repeat this exercise routine for four consecutive weeks

I highly recommend you SLOWLY ease into the movement of each exercise and allow your body to get used to the intensity and body positioning carefully.

Injuries happen from moving too fast during exercise as well as from performing new exercises. Be mindful of both of these facts and use this knowledge to guide how hard you push yourself in each movement.

The goal here is to apply slow and concentrated contractions to the targeted areas and allow them to respond by growing stronger.

Taking a day of rest from the exercises is almost as important as performing the exercises themselves.

This day off from the workout will allow your body the 24-48 hours it needs to ADAPT and grow stronger.

Stress…adapt…stress…adapt…

The Exercises are as follows:

- The Flying Super Senior
- Abdominal Hold
- Squat
- Seated Chair Pulls
- Outward Shoulder Press
- Kneeling Push Ups
- Hip Lifts

One of the most simple and effective exercises you can do at home to strengthen the lower back muscles can be done the moment you wake up in the morning. This movement, as with all of the following exercises in this book is designed to specifically target each major muscle group. The Flying Super Senior Exercise is one is the most difficult to learn, but after only a few workouts. You will become MUCH stronger on the backside of your body. This exercise may help you if you are having lower back pain.

Because of its importance, I call this exercise the:

"Flying Super Senior."

(Imagine the guy who wears the red cape.) ☺

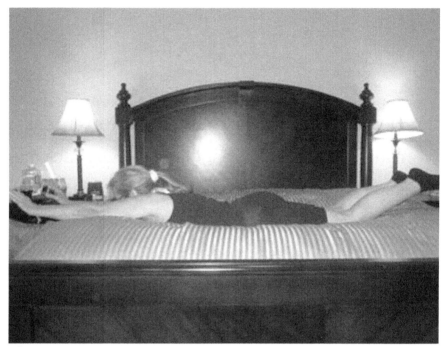

Flying Super Senior Exercise

The **Flying Super Senior** is performed lying face down in bed, with your head being supported by a small pillow. Place your arms straight out and point them toward your headboard. Next, place your feet together with your feet hanging off the end of your bed.

It is important to only involve raising your head off the pillow if and when you have fairly strong neck muscles because it could cause neck strain or discomfort. If you have even the slightest bit of chance that you may have weak neck muscles, or you want to be a little more cautious about the strengthening process, do this:
After you perform this exercise for the first week, slowly begin adding the lifting of your head into the exercise. DO this very slowly and do not over-exert your neck muscles.

Raise your limbs first, then slowly raise your head the slightest amount, let the muscles begin to activate and start to become fatigued and STOP before letting this exercise become too difficult on these muscles.

Hold this contracted position (as contracted as YOU feel comfortable with) as long as you can hold this movement one time for each workout.

Do one of these body position "holds" and then move on to the next exercise.

By the second or third week, you should be able to lift the head in unison with the limbs and you should be starting to feel…well…SUPER!

Strengthen these muscles SLOWLY, but keep in mind that they are muscles and that they need to be carefully pushed to cause a safe amount of fatigue, accordingly. Otherwise no strength increase will occur.

It is also important to keep in mind that if you feel any pain throughout any of these exercises, you should terminate the exercise immediately and consult your physician.

Your goal here is to engage in the exercise lifting your hands and feet only ONE INCH or even less, in order to activate not only the muscles of the lower back. Performing the Flying Super Senior will also send a signal to all of the muscles on the backside of your body. This signal will tell them they need to respond and that they must ADAPT by growing stronger.

Note: Please read the Summary of the Flying Super Senior below. It is extremely important you have a full grasp of how to perform each exercise safely and SLOWLY in order to not only avoid injury, but to also receive the greatest benefits.

*Before doing these exercises please consult your physician to ensure you are cleared for this type of activity. If at any point during any of these exercises you feel any pain, stop the exercise immediately and consult your physician.

A Summary of how to perform this exercise properly…

- Begin by lying on your stomach with your feet together and your arms stretched out, forward of your head.

- Very slowly raise your arms off of the bed approximately 1 inch. Do the same with your legs.

CAUTION: Beginners (or those who may be considered very weak) should begin this movement by, NOT lifting their arms and legs, but by engaging these muscles AS IF to lift your arms and legs into the air, but stopping short of raising your limbs.

Beginner's Note: Your arms and legs DO NOT actually come up off the mattress.

After the first few exercise sessions, you should be able to add the lifting of your limbs to this exercise as a means of adding the resistance you soon will require!

Simply by engaging these muscle groups and HOLDING for as long as possible, you will become stronger and soon, if enough rest is allowed between exercise sessions. As you grow stronger, you should soon be able to move your hands and feet into the "one inch" position.

This exercise is performed for as long as you can "hold" this position. This position will act as a trigger, and can cause these muscle groups to grow stronger.

Beginner's Note: A Beginner variation for the Flying Super Senior is to alternate lifting one leg with the opposing arm. See below:

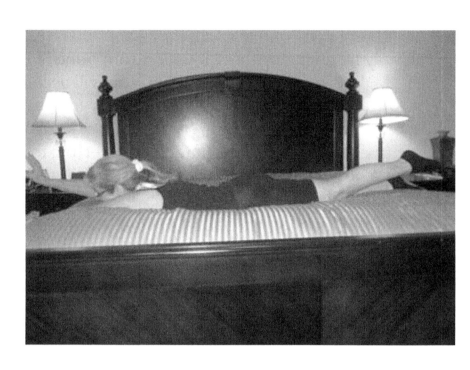

Once you have done the Flying Super Senior exercise, you will then proceed to the next exercise. The next exercise will begin to strengthen the front part of your abdominal muscles (Stomach) and the front upper leg muscles. (Thighs)

The next thing you need to do, after completing the Flying Super Senior is simply ROLL OVER.

Abdominals & Front Thighs

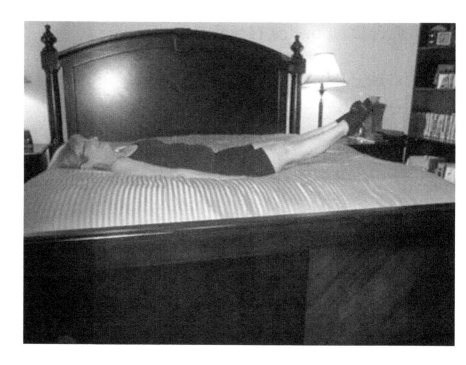

How to perform this exercise:

The second exercise is performed in a position lying on your back with your arms stretched overhead. One should keep their legs together. This is a very similar starting position as the Super Senior exercise.

Position your arms straight down by your side, with your palms pressed against the bed to stabilize the body.
With your feet together, lift your legs slowly 1-6 inches off of the bed. While holding your legs in this position, SLOWLY press down with the palms of your hands, against the mattress.

Keep your arms straight. When performed correctly, you will feel the muscles of the thighs and stomach muscles contract. This exercise activates the front torso muscles, also known as your "core" muscles. This area is extremely important for stabilization of your body.

After a few workouts, or if you're a stronger trainee, you may stretch your arms over your head and lift your arms and legs at the same time, only allowing them to come up a couple of inches off the bed.

Continue creating slowly throughout the duration of this exercise. Stop immediately if you feel any pain. Slowly, let your body get used to these movements.

The objective again here is to tax these muscles safely and in a controlled manner, and give them a signal that the most indeed grow stronger. Hold each pose as long as comfortably possible.

Never hold your breath, and always breathe normally and maintain correct form. Maintaining form in every exercise is crucial to minimize the risk of injury and also to minimize the involvement of this sensitive neck muscles and other muscles that are not intended to be involved in each exercise.

Beginner's Note:

As with the Flying Super Senior exercise, beginners may want to start off with one leg for the first few workouts and then add the second leg as they gain in strength, from the previous exercise sessions.

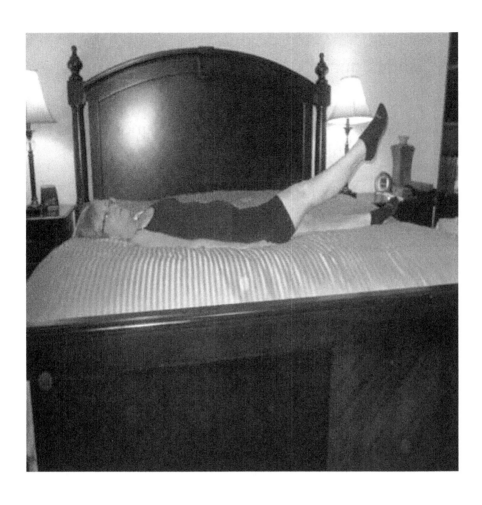

Body Squats

This exercise can be performed standing next to a kitchen table or kitchen counter. (See Below)

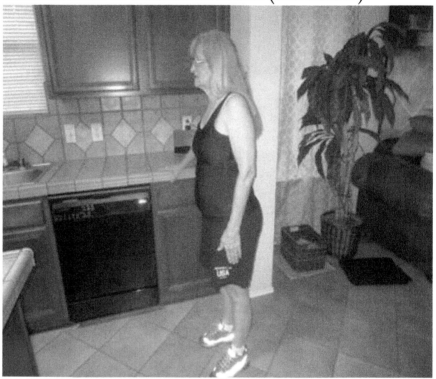

Starting Position

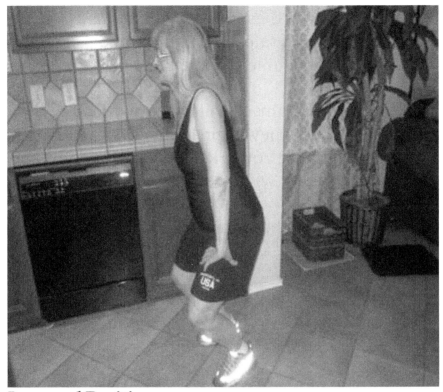

Lowered Position

Exercise Description:
Begin this exercise standing next to a counter, or table.
Place your feet should-width apart.
Stand up straight.
Look forward and slowly bend your knees and lower your body as low as you feel comfortable. Pretend you are going to sit in a chair.
Slowly return to the top position.

Do as many of these SLOW repetitions as you can until you feel a safe, but slight "fatigue" feeling throughout your legs and glutes.

*Note: Most trainees will look down during this exercise, or as they begin to tire. Do NOT do this. This may cause you to lean forward and you should remain upright while performing this exercise.

Look straight ahead throughout the duration of the exercise.

This helps to keep the back straight.

The next exercise:

The Seated Arm Pulls

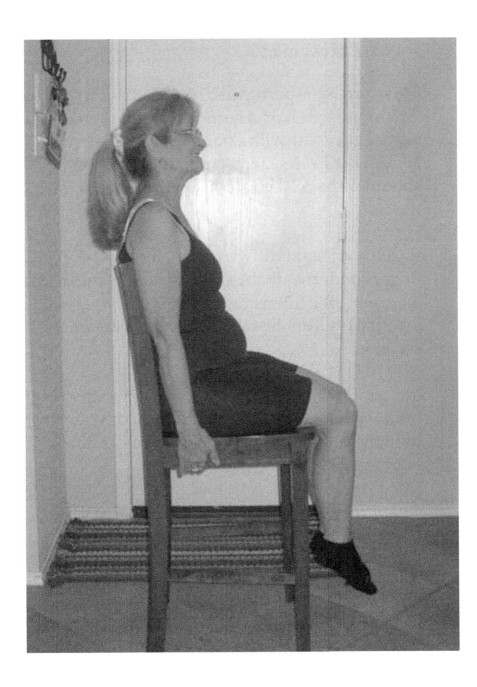

Exercise Movement:

This exercise is performed seated upright in a chair. Any standard chair is sufficient. Start the exercise seated in a chair with your back pressed firmly against the back seat rest, posture straight up shoulders back. It is important to maintain this posture.

Reach both hands down next to the hips, curl your fingers underneath the seat and slowly pull upward, increasing the intensity. Maintain a slow and steady upward pull, against the bottom of the seat, for 10 seconds.

In your first few routines, do not pull with maximum force. Resist the urge to pull with all of your strength until the muscles get stronger (usually after only your first few workouts.)

Again, pull upwards with the hands while maintaining perfect posture, for ten seconds.

At the end of ten seconds, terminate this exercise.

Outward Shoulder Press

This exercise is performed standing in a doorway.

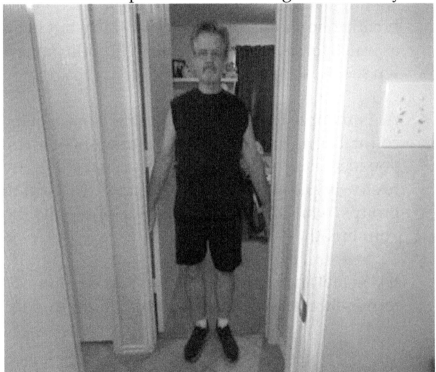

Outward Shoulder Press

Place the outsides of your hands firmly against the door jams as shown in the picture.
While keeping a straight back, you should look up and slowly apply pressure (outwards) against the door jams.

Carefully apply as much force as comfortably possible for a period of ten seconds.

After ten seconds, terminate the set.

Again **posture is very important**. Do not hold your breath; one should breathe comfortably but maintain as much force as possible against the door jams for ten seconds.

As you apply force against the door jams, slowly count to ten. Try to increase the amount of force as you increase your count. Once again the objective is to slowly and safely apply pressure to these muscle groups, while not sacrificing good form or holding your breath.

If you feel any pain during this exercise, immediately terminate the exercise and consult your physician.

Kneeling Push Ups

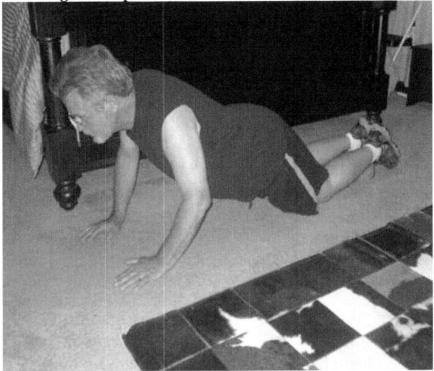

Kneeling Push Up

The next exercise is similar to the Push Up.

For advanced trainees or stronger women and men, you can perform this exercise from your feet and perform a standard variation of push up. (The kneeling variation is pictured).

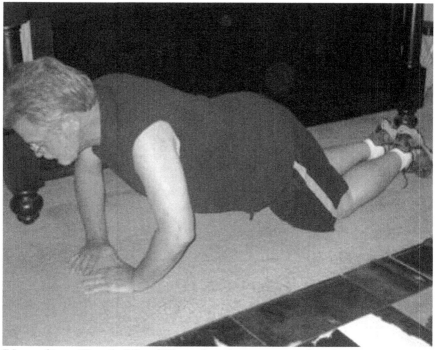

Kneeling Push Up (Hands close together)

A closer hand position will target more of the area located on the back of the arms.

A wider hand position targets the chest and shoulders in a more focused manner.

The exercise is performed as follows:

Begin in the upper position and slowly lower your upper body down approximately 4-6 inches. Then press back up.
Maintain a slight bend in your elbows at the top of the exercise and do a smooth turnaround at both the top and bottom positions.

One should only allow your upper body to travel HALFWAY down to the floor, at its lowest point. Then push back up.

Repeat this motion up and down until you develop fatigue in the muscles.

The objective here is to tax the muscles without causing strain. You will have to be your own judge based on your current level of strength.

Keep in mind that with all of these exercises, the further you SAFELY push yourself to muscular fatigue in each one, the more of a signal you will have sent to each corresponding muscle group to GET STRONGER.

Never sacrifice good posture and form in an attempt to try harder.

No matter how difficult the exercises becomes...**NEVER hold your breath**.

Breathe naturally.

SAFETY FIRST!

Hip Lifts

Starting Position

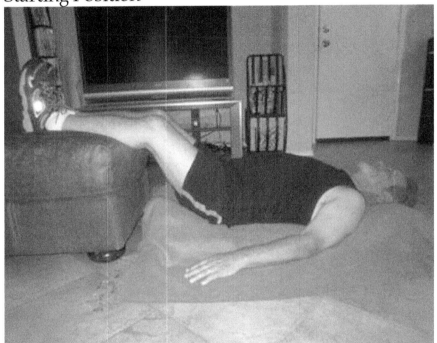

Hip Lifts

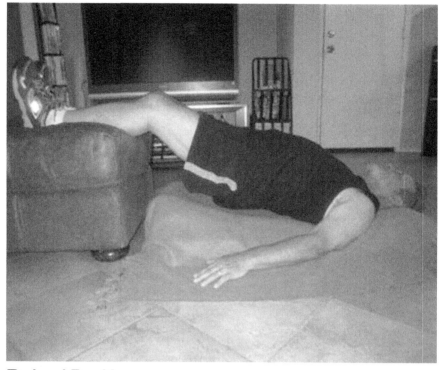

Raised Position

Exercise Description:

Begin this exercise lying on the floor, with your legs raised onto a chair or ottoman. (As shown above).

Place your palms down by your side and slowly lift your pelvis up in the air.

This will cause your glutes and the back of your legs to do the work. Lift as high as is comfortable FOR YOU.

Do as many lifts as comfortably possible.

You are your best guide and let the slow feeling of muscle contraction be your guide.

After the first week of exercising you should have a very comfortable grasp of how to safely position yourself into each exercise. Remember, you will avoid most injury by going slow and testing your own body's current level of existing strength and adjust the exercise intensity accordingly.

When in doubt, STOP, re-examine your form and try the exercise again.

Practice makes better!

Exercise Plan Summary:

- **The Flying Super Senior** – Hold as long as comfortably possible
- **Abdominal Hold** – Hold as long as comfortably possible
- **Squats** – Do as many as you can without over exerting yourself
- **Seated Chair Pulls** – Hold for 10 seconds
- **Outward Shoulder Press** – Hold for 10 seconds
- **Kneeling Push Ups** - Do as many as you comfortably can

- **Hip Lifts** - Hold as long as comfortably possible

Walking

Walking is one of the most important activities you can do for your body. Walking burns almost as many calories as running but does not subject your joints and tendons to the pounding of running.

Walking is great for your mind and body. Even if you have to walk slowly and if only for a few minutes each day, do it. This activity is crucial to keep your hips, joints and vertebrae moving together in alignment (unless you have an injury) and just this simple act of moving each day will slowly build up your strength in your lower back, hips and knees.

When you have to deal with hot or cold weather outside, try walking early in the morning, after your cup of coffee. Another alternative is to walk at night if possible. If you have access to a treadmill, this should become your new best friend.

Try to walk a little bit each day. Walking keeps your vertebrae strong, burns calories and best of all...

It's FREE and it's FUN!

The exercises in this e-book, when performed correctly, have proven to increase strength and mobility throughout the major muscle groups of the body. Your results happen very quickly from this cause-and-effect training. Remember, this is an exercise SCIENCE and it is based upon the fundamental, physiological systems of the human body.

In weaker trainees (or for people who may only be weak in these specific muscle groups) the resulting strength gains can happen overnight!

These exercises should all be performed during the same routine. Most trainees will experience a considerable increase in strength, from only the first few workouts. You will begin to notice this increase in strength throughout the course of your daily activities.

Many people experience not only a reduction of muscular and joint pain after only just a few workouts, but also find that they sleep better throughout the night.

This is mainly because of the demand that the exercises place upon your muscles and central nervous system.

What you're doing in this routine is literally sending signals to the self-preservation system of the body and **ordering it too grow stronger.**

Here is a bit more about what makes this routine so effective in improving your strength vs. the less-effective routines suggested by many exercise books

•   Pay close attention to the exercises that are supposed to be held for 10 seconds, as opposed to the ones in which you need to hold for as long as possible.

- The reason is, the exercises with added resistance (chair, wall, etc.) allow you to flip your muscle's "strength switch" in a matter of seconds, providing you are applying enough force. The others require more time.

- The other exercises require you to hold the pose because (a) when there is no resistance, you NEED to give your body a reason to become stronger and holding as long as possible will do that and (b) doing some arbitrary number of repetitions (like 10) will do almost NOTHING to improve your strength (after maybe one or two weeks) while the manner in which I have you perform these exercises, literally forces your body to become stronger from every single workout, provided you gave the routine enough effort. .

- **The method of performing these techniques, the force (intensity) by which you apply pressure to stationary objects and the constantly increasing "hold time" for the flying super senior are some of the most important aspects of this routine. These are the fundamental factors, which will cause your muscles to become stronger. Remember this.**

Conclusion

If you like this book, please tell a friend or family member.

It is my hope that together, by motivating each other and sharing these simple but effective exercises and techniques, we can help improve the lives of as many of our wonderful seniors as possible.

A rising tide lifts all boats.

Carpe' Diem,

Kevin Saint Clair

"Age wrinkles the body,
Quitting wrinkles the soul."
-General Douglas MacArthur

About The Author:

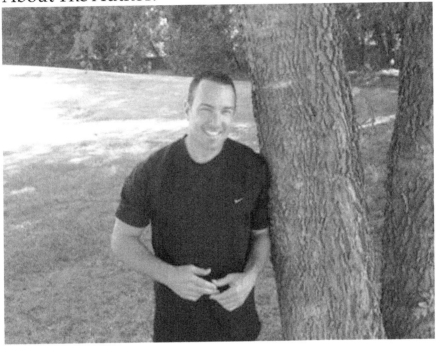

Kevin Saint Clair developed a passion for how the muscles of the human body function as a teenager. In addition to spending many years traveling internationally, he has spent more than 20 years studying the relationship between our muscles and the central nervous system.

As both a passion and a hobby…

Kevin has trained champion athletes, military personnel and designed strength training programs for sports teams.

Kevin's mission is to help improve the quality-of-life of others.

Models:
Richard and Cecilia

In addition to being wonderful people and kind enough to model for this book, Richard is also a **licensed occupational therapist** and Cecilia is a **residential home sales agent** in Texas.

Thank you for your assistance!

Made in the USA
Middletown, DE
23 April 2021